Copyright ©

All rights reserv

may be reproduced, distributed, or transmitted in any form or by any means, including photocopying, recording, or other electronic or mechanical methods, without the prior written permission of the publisher, except in the case of brief quotations embodied in critical reviews and certain other noncommercial uses permitted by copyright law

Table of Contents

Introduction..5

Diet details..6

A new healthy diet 14

Single Serving Recipes You Need in Your Bariatric Life 19

Chicken, Bacon and Ranch Wonton Cupcakes.........22

Sesame Chicken Wonton Cups 25

Meatloaf Muffin with Mashed Potato Frosting 29

Chicken Broccoli Alfredo Wonton Cupcakes 32

Skinny Meatloaf Muffins with BBQ Sauce...............35

Crunchy Taco Cups 38

Chicken Cordon Bleu Wonton Cupcakes 41

Crab Salad in Crisp Wonton Cup...........................44

Thai Chicken Salad Wonton Cups 47

Buffalo Chicken Cups..................................51

Boom Bang-a-Bang Chicken Cups........................54

Ancho Chile Ground Beef Tacos........................56

Garlic Lemon Shrimp Kabobs...........................59

Pumpkin Pie Oatmeal (with Added Protein) 61

BBQ Breakfast Chicken Burritos.......................63

Chunky Unstuffed Green Peppers 65

Slow Cooker Creamy Italian Chicken...................66

Slow Cooker Salsa Chicken with Cheese Soup..........68

Breaded Chicken Parmesan.............................70

Slow-Cooker Salsa Chicken 71

Grape Salad..72

Grape Salad..74

Slow Cooker Chicken Taco Stew 75

Chock Full O' Flavor Chicken Salad 77

Chock Full O' Flavor Chicken Salad 78

Amy's Mexican Chicken Casserole...........................78

Chicken Salad 81

Chicken & Grape Salad 83

Meal Plan for Steady Weight Loss (1 Week Plan)........84

The Bottom Line...99

Introduction

A gastric bypass diet helps people who are recovering from sleeve gastrectomy and from gastric bypass surgery also known as Roux-en-Y gastric bypass to heal and to change their eating habits.

As a registered dietitian, I have explained in this book about the diet you'll need to follow after surgery, explaining what types of food and how much you can eat at each meal. Closely following your gastric bypass diet can help you lose weight safely.

Purpose

The gastric bypass diet is designed to:

- Allow your stomach to heal without being stretched by the food you eat

- Get you used to eating the smaller amounts of food that your smaller stomach can comfortably and safely digest
- Help you lose weight and avoid gaining weight
- Avoid side effects and complications from the surgery

Diet details

Diet recommendations after gastric bypass surgery vary depending on your individual situation.

A gastric bypass diet typically follows a staged approach to help you ease back into eating solid foods. How quickly you move from one step to the next depends on how fast your body heals and adjusts to the change in eating patterns. You can usually start eating regular foods about three months after surgery.

At each stage of the gastric bypass diet, you must be careful to:

- Drink 64 ounces of fluid a day, to avoid dehydration.

- Sip liquids between meals, not with meals. Wait about 30 minutes after a meal to drink anything and avoid drinking 30 minutes before a meal.

- Eat and drink slowly, to avoid dumping syndrome — which occurs when foods and liquids enter your small intestine rapidly and in larger amounts than normal, causing nausea, vomiting, dizziness, sweating and diarrhea.

- Eat lean, protein-rich foods daily.

- Choose foods and drinks that are low in fats and sugar.

- Avoid alcohol.

- Limit caffeine, which can cause dehydration.

- Take vitamin and mineral supplements daily as directed by your health provider.

- Chew foods thoroughly to a pureed consistency before swallowing, once you progress beyond liquids only.

Liquids

For the first day or so after surgery, you'll only be allowed to drink clear liquids. Once you're handling clear liquids, you can start having other liquids, such as:

- Broth

- Unsweetened juice

- Decaffeinated tea or coffee

- Milk (skim or 1 percent)

- Sugar-free gelatin or popsicles

Pureed foods

After about a week of tolerating liquids, you can begin to eat strained and pureed (mashed up) foods. The foods should have the consistency of a smooth paste or a thick liquid, without any solid pieces of food in the mixture.

You can eat three to six small meals a day. Each meal should consist of 4 to 6 tablespoons of food. Eat slowly, about 30 minutes for each meal.

Choose foods that will puree well, such as:

- Lean ground meat, poultry or fish

- Cottage cheese

- Soft scrambled eggs

- Cooked cereal

- Soft fruits and cooked vegetables

- Strained cream soups

Blend solid foods with a liquid, such as:

- Water

- Skim milk

- Juice with no sugar added

- Broth

Soft foods

After a few weeks of pureed foods, and with your doctor's OK, you can add soft foods to your diet. They should be small, tender and easily chewed pieces of food.

You can eat three to five small meals a day. Each meal should consist of one-third to one-half cup of food. Chew each bite until the food is pureed consistency before swallowing.

Soft foods include:

- Ground lean meat or poultry
- Flaked fish
- Eggs
- Cottage cheese
- Cooked or dried cereal
- Rice

- Canned or soft fresh fruit, without seeds or skin

- Cooked vegetables, without skin

Solid foods

After about eight weeks on the gastric bypass diet, you can gradually return to eating firmer foods. Start with eating three meals a day, with each meal consisting of 1 to 1-1/2 cups of food. It's important to stop eating before you feel completely full.

Depending on how you tolerate solid food, you may be able to vary the number of meals and amount of food at each meal. Talk to your dietitian about what's best for you.

Try new foods one at a time. Certain foods may cause pain, nausea or vomiting after gastric bypass surgery.

Foods that can cause problems at this stage include:

- Breads

- Carbonated drinks

- Raw vegetables

- Cooked fibrous vegetables, such as celery, broccoli, corn or cabbage

- Tough meats or meats with gristle

- Red meat

- Fried foods

- Highly seasoned or spicy foods

- Nuts and seeds

- Popcorn

Over time, you might be able to try some of these foods again, with the guidance of your doctor.

A new healthy diet

Gastric bypass surgery reduces the size of your stomach and changes the way food enters your intestines. After surgery, it's important to get adequate nourishment while keeping your weight-loss goals on track. Your doctor is likely to recommend that you:

- Eat and drink slowly. To avoid dumping syndrome, take at least 30 minutes to eat your meals and 30 to 60 minutes to drink 1 cup of liquid. Wait 30 minutes before or after each meal to drink liquids.
- Keep meals small. Eat several small meals a day. You might start with six small meals a day, then move to four meals and finally, when following a regular diet, three meals a day. Each meal should include about a half-cup to 1 cup of food.

- Drink liquids between meals. To avoid dehydration, you'll need to drink at least 8 cups (1.9 liters) of fluids a day. But drinking too much liquid at or around mealtime can leave you feeling overly full and prevent you from eating enough nutrient-rich food.

- Chew food thoroughly. The new opening that leads from your stomach into your small intestine is very narrow and can be blocked by larger pieces of food. Blockages prevent food from leaving your stomach and can cause vomiting, nausea and abdominal pain. Take small bites of food and chew them to a pureed consistency before swallowing.

- Focus on high-protein foods. Eat these foods before you eat other foods in your meal.

- Avoid foods that are high in fat and sugar. These foods travel quickly through your digestive system and cause dumping syndrome.

- Take recommended vitamin and mineral supplements. After surgery your body won't be able to absorb enough nutrients from your food. You'll likely need to take a multivitamin supplement every day for the rest of your life.

Results

The gastric bypass diet can help you recover from surgery and transition to a way of eating that is healthy and supports your weight-loss goals. Remember that if you return to unhealthy eating habits after weight-loss surgery, you may not lose all of your excess weight, or you may regain any weight that you do lose.

Risks

The greatest risks of the gastric bypass diet come from not following the diet properly. If you eat too much or eat food that you shouldn't, you could have complications. These include:

- Dumping syndrome. If too much food enters your small intestine quickly, you are likely to experience nausea, vomiting, dizziness, sweating and diarrhea. Eating too much or too fast, eating foods high in fat or sugar, and not chewing your food adequately can all cause nausea or vomiting after meals.

- Dehydration. Because you're not supposed to drink fluids with your meals, some people become dehydrated. That's why you need to sip 64 ounces (1.9 liters) of water and other fluids throughout the day.

- Constipation. A lack of physical activity and of fiber or fluid in your diet can cause constipation.

- Blocked opening of your stomach pouch. Food can become lodged at the opening of your stomach pouch, even if you carefully follow the diet. Signs and symptoms of a blocked stomach opening include ongoing nausea, vomiting and abdominal pain. Call your doctor if you have these symptoms for more than two days.

- Weight gain or failure to lose weight. If you continue to gain weight or fail to lose weight on the gastric bypass diet, talk to your doctor or dietitian.

Single Serving Recipes You Need in Your Bariatric Life

Planning healthy meals that work with your bariatric diet can be tough. You need these bariatric recipes in your life!

Traditionally we find ourselves in one of these two boats:

- Tasty, but unhealthy OR
- Healthy, but not tasty

Try our alternative: Tasty and healthy

Have your bariatric meals left you unsatisfied? The dietary restriction that comes with being a bariatric patient can be frustrating to put it lightly. What if you didn't have to sacrifice the foods you love or your weight loss progress?

At it's most basic level, weight loss is a numbers game. If we are regularly in a calorie surplus (consuming more calories than our bodies burn) we gain weight, if we eat fewer calories than we burn we lose weight. It really is that simple. Then why can it be so hard to lose weight on a consistent basis?

Effective meal preparation and portion control solve this problem altogether. If you want guilt-free, delicious and portion-controlled meals that work with any meal plan you need to try these recipes!

Get exactly the nutrition you need, in exactly the serving sizes you need

One thing that makes cooking in bulk or one-pot recipes (like in a crockpot or a casserole) difficult for meal-planning is that the number of servings isn't exact. Calculating the calories per serving requires busting out a spreadsheet just to get your calories and macro numbers. Then you have to measure that quantity out every time you get a serving. Not ideal.

Each recipe in this book yields individually packaged single servings, which makes portion control as simple as it can be. You can make an entire batch and save the rest for days and enjoy stress-free, delicious meal-planning.

Chicken, Bacon and Ranch Wonton Cupcakes

This recipe brings all of your favorite flavors together in a tight, organized package. Who says you can't enjoy the perfectly married flavor of bacon and ranch while losing weight? Light ranch seasoning, bacon and lean chicken breast make this an unbeatable option for healthy eating. Makes 12 Wonton Cups.

NUTRITION INFORMATION PER CUP:

152 calories | 10 g carbs | 6 g fat | 14 g protein

INGREDIENTS

1 lb uncooked boneless, skinless chicken breasts

- 1 tablespoon ranch seasoning

- 2 teaspoons canola oil

- 5 slices center cut bacon, cooked crisp and chopped

- ¾ cup yogurt-based ranch dressing (such as Bolthouse Farms)
- 24 wonton wrappers
- 4 oz 2% shredded sharp cheddar

DIRECTIONS:

1. Preheat the oven to 375. Lightly mist 12 cups in a standard muffin/cupcake tin with cooking spray and set aside.
2. Place the uncooked chicken strips into a Ziploc bag and sprinkle with the ranch seasoning. Seal the bag and shake/massage until the chicken is coated with the seasoning.
3. Bring the canola oil over medium heat in a medium-sized skillet. When the oil is hot, add the

chicken pieces and stir them around to coat with oil. Arrange them into a single layer and cook for 5-7 minutes, flipping occasionally, until the chicken strips are cooked through. Remove the chicken to a cutting board and chop into small pieces.

4. Place the chopped chicken into a mixing bowl and stir in the chopped bacon and ranch dressing until well combined.

5. Push a wonton wrapper into the bottom of each of the sprayed cups in the muffin tin. Using about half of the chicken mixture, spoon evenly into the wonton wrappers. Sprinkle about half of the shredded cheddar evenly over the top of each cup. Press another wonton wrapper on top and repeat the layering steps with the remaining chicken mixture and shredded cheddar.

6. Bake for 18-20 minutes until the wontons are golden brown and the contents are heated through. Remove the muffin tin from the oven and allow to cool for 2-3 minutes before removing from the tin

Sesame Chicken Wonton Cups

If Asian fusion in a crispy package isn't enough to get you excited then we have a bigger problem on our hands. Chicken doesn't have to be boring and bland. Don't forget the sesame seeds and the cilantro to really make this one stand out! Makes 24 Wonton Cups.

NUTRITION INFORMATION PER CUPCAKE:

152 calories | 10 g carbs | 6 g fat | 14 g protein

INGREDIENTS

- 8 ounces boneless, skinless chicken breast

- cooking spray

- 24 wonton wrappers, about 6 oz.

- 2 tablespoons tahini

- 2 tablespoons soy sauce or tamari sauce

- 2 tablespoons maple syrup

- 2 tablespoons mayonnaise

- ½ cup thinly sliced snow peas

- ½ cup shredded carrot

- ½ cup thinly sliced scallions

- 2 tablespoons chopped basil and/or cilantro

- black sesame seeds for garnish, optional

DIRECTIONS:

1. Place chicken breast in a medium skillet and cover with cold tap water. Place over high heat and bring to a simmer. Reduce heat to maintain a gentle simmer and cook until the chicken is no longer pink in the center and cooked through, 8 to 12 minutes, depending on thickness of the meat. Remove the chicken and let cool. Cut chicken into small cubes.

2. Meanwhile, Preheat oven to 350°F. Coat two 12-cup mini-muffin tins with cooking spray. Cut corners off wonton wrappers to make an octagonal shape. Gently press wrapper down into each cup. Lightly spritz wrappers with cooking spray.

3. Transfer the pans to the oven and bake until the wrappers are starting to turn golden brown and are

crispy and bubbling, 10 to 14 minutes. Let cool completely.

4. Whisk tahini, soy or tamari, maple syrup and mayonnaise in a medium bowl until smooth. Stir in the chicken and refrigerate until cold, 40 minutes to 1 hour.

5. Stir snow peas, carrots, scallions and herbs into chicken mixture. Divide chicken salad among wonton cups, about 2 scant tablespoons each. Garnish with sesame seeds, if using. Serve immediately.

Meatloaf Muffin with Mashed Potato Frosting

While this one is a different play on the cup-cake you must give it a chance. If you like the staple of meatloaf and mashed potatoes you'll love every perfect bite of this healthy pairing. Use lean ground beef or turkey (at least 93% lean) and you can fit this into any diet. Makes 12 Cupcakes.

NUTRITION INFORMATION PER CUPCAKE:

120 calories | 12.25 g carbs | 4.25 g fat | 9 g protein

INGREDIENTS

For the Meatloaf Cupcakes:

- 1.3 lb 93% lean ground turkey
- 1 cup grated zucchini, all moisture squeezed dry with paper towel
- 2 tbsp onion, minced

- 1/2 cup seasoned breadcrumbs

- 1/4 cup ketchup

- 1 egg

- 1 tsp kosher salt

For the Skinny Mashed Potato "Frosting":

- 1 lb (about 2 medium) Yukon gold potatoes, peeled and cubed

- 2 large garlic cloves, peeled and halved

- 2 tbsp fat free sour cream

- 2 tbsp fat free chicken broth

- 1 tbsp skim milk

- 1/2 tbsp light butter

- kosher salt to taste

- dash of fresh ground pepper

- 2 tbsp fresh thyme

DIRECTIONS:

1. Put the potatoes and garlic in a large pot with salt and enough water to cover; bring to a boil.

2. Cover and reduce heat; simmer for 20 minutes or until potatoes are tender.

3. Drain and return potatoes and garlic to pan. Add sour cream and remaining ingredients.

4. Using a masher or blender, mash until smooth.

5. Season with salt and pepper to taste.

6. Meanwhile, preheat the oven to 350°.

7. Line a muffin tin with foil liners.

8. In a large bowl, mix the turkey, zucchini, onion, breadcrumbs, ketchup, egg, and salt.

9. Place meatloaf mixture into muffin tins, filling them to the top, making sure they are flat at the top.

10. Bake uncovered for 18-20 minutes or until cooked through.

11. Remove from tins and place onto a baking dish.

12. Pipe the "frosting" onto the meatloaf cupcakes and serve.

Chicken Broccoli Alfredo Wonton Cupcakes

When you want a healthy meal it normally won't include creamy Alfredo at any capacity. Luckily you're reading this recipe and will love how it can fit easily into your bariatric diet whether you are maintaining your current weight or are still on your journey to your goal weight. The Italian seasoning and light Alfredo sauce makes this feel like a cheat meal, you will come back to this one many times! Makes 12 Cups.

NUTRITION INFORMATION PER CUP:

130 calories | 9 g carbs | 5 g fat | 13 g protein

INGREDIENTS

- 1 ½ teaspoons olive oil
- 1 cup broccoli florets, chopped small
- 2 cups cooked shredded or diced chicken breast
- 1 cup light Alfredo sauce
- ½ teaspoon Italian seasoning
- 1/8 teaspoon black pepper
- 24 wonton wrappers
- 1 ½ cup shredded 2% Mozzarella cheese
- 1 tablespoon grated Parmesan cheese

DIRECTIONS:

1. Pre-heat the oven to 375. Lightly mist 12 cups in a standard muffin/cupcake tin with cooking spray and set aside.

2. Pour the oil into a skillet and bring over medium heat. Add the broccoli and cook for 5 minutes or until broccoli is tender, stirring occasionally.

3. Transfer the broccoli to a mixing bowl and combine with the chicken, alfredo sauce, Italian seasoning and pepper. Stir until well combined.

4. Push a wonton wrapper into the bottom of each of the sprayed cups in the muffin tin. Using about half of the chicken mixture, spoon evenly into the wonton wrappers. Sprinkle about half the Mozzarella cheese evenly over the top of each cup. Press another wonton wrapper on top and repeat

the layering steps with the remaining chicken mixture and Mozzarella cheese. When complete, sprinkle ¼ teaspoon of Parmesan cheese over the top of each wonton cup.

5. Bake for 18-20 minutes until golden brown.

Skinny Meatloaf Muffins with BBQ Sauce

This one is just in time for summer! No need to kick the bbq for good when options like these delicious muffins are in the cards. Using lean turkey or ground beef makes it a no-brainer for the health-conscious and the foodie alike. Don't skimp on the Worcestershire sauce and experiment with different bbq sauces! Makes 9 Servings.

NUTRITION INFORMATION PER CUP:

115 calories | 18 g carbs | 2 g fat | 18 g protein

INGREDIENTS

- 1 package (~1.25 pounds) 99% fat-free ground turkey breast
- ½ cup bread crumbs
- 1 cup onions, finely diced
- 1 egg
- 2 tablespoons Worcestershire sauce
- ½ cup barbecue
- ¼ teaspoon salt
- Fresh ground pepper, to taste

DIRECTIONS:

1. Preheat oven to 350 degrees. Coat a regular (12-cup) muffin pan with cooking spray. Since this

recipe makes 9 meatloaf muffins, you'll only fill 9 not 12. Set aside.

2. To make bread crumbs: Toast 1 slice whole wheat or multigrain bread. Place in a blender and pulse until made into crumbs.

3. In a large bowl, add ground turkey, bread crumbs, onions, egg, Worcestershire sauce, ½ cup barbecue sauce, salt and pepper. Using your hands or a large spoon, thoroughly mix together until well blended.

4. Add meatloaf mixture to the 9 muffin cups, flattening out the tops. Top each meatloaf muffin with ¾ tablespoon barbecue sauce and spread evenly over top.

5. Bake for 40 minutes. Run a knife around each muffin to loosen it from pan. Remove to a serving plate.

Crunchy Taco Cups

Mexican food is normally packed with cheese, cream and unnecessary fats. These traditionally calorie dense choices lead to blissful overeating. If you make these taco cups you'll get the best of both worlds: delicious, south-of-the-boarder taste without the guilt that normally follows! We like reduced sodium taco seasoning. It tastes just as good and it's best to avoid excessive sodium when we can. If you are feeling "fancy," substitute the Rotel tomatoes with some freshly diced tomatoes. The fresh tomatoes and thin layer of melted cheese makes this an instant classic. Makes 12 Taco Cups.

NUTRITION INFORMATION PER CUP:

178 calories | 10.4 g carbs | 7.3 g fat | 16.8 g protein

INGREDIENTS

- 1 lb lean ground beef, browned and drained
- 1 envelope (3 tablespoons) taco seasoning
- 1 (10-oz) can Ro-Tel Diced Tomatoes and Green Chiles
- 1½ cups sharp cheddar cheese, shredded (or Mexican blend)
- 24 wonton wrappers

DIRECTIONS:

1. Preheat oven to 375 degrees F. Generously coat a standard size muffin tin with nonstick cooking spray.

2. Combine cooked beef, taco seasoning, and tomatoes in a bowl and stir to combine. Line each cup of the prepared muffin tin with a wonton wrapper. Add 1.5 tablespoons taco mixture. Top with 1 tablespoon of cheese. Press down and add another layer of wonton wrapper, taco mixture, and a final layer of cheese.

3. Bake at 375 for 11-13 minutes until cups are heated through and edges are golden.

Chicken Cordon Bleu Wonton Cupcakes

Chicken Cordon Bleu may make you think of a generic banquet hall buffet, but give this a try and you'll have a change of heart. One thing that Chicken Cordon Blue has gotten right is the combination of smooth cheese and delicious ham paired with lean, healthy chicken. Those aspects aren't lost here in this perfect "cupcake." Makes 12 "Cupcakes.

NUTRITION INFORMATION PER CUP:

152 calories | 10 g carbs | 4 g fat | 17 g protein

INGREDIENTS

- 12 oz (2 ½ cups) cooked diced or shredded chicken breast
- 3 oz thinly sliced deli ham, chopped

- 8 wedges of The Laughing Cow Light Swiss Cheese Wedges, chopped
- 1 teaspoon mustard
- 24 wonton wrappers
- 6 slices 2% Swiss Cheese, each cut into 4 equal pieces
- 0.75 oz seasoned croutons, crushed

DIRECTIONS:

1. Pre-heat the oven to 375. Lightly mist 12 cups in a standard muffin/cupcake tin with cooking spray and set aside.

2. In a microwave-safe mixing bowl, combine the chicken, ham, chopped cheese wedges and mustard and stir together. Place the bowl in the

microwave and heat on high for 1 ½ minutes until contents are warm. Use a spoon to mix contents and smush the cheese wedges until they've coated the meat.

3. Push a wonton wrapper into the bottom of each of the sprayed cups in the muffin tin. Using about half of the chicken mixture, spoon evenly into the wonton wrappers. Place one of the 2% Swiss pieces on top of each cup. Press another wonton wrapper on top and repeat the layering steps with the remaining chicken mixture and 2% Swiss cheese.

4. Bake for 10 minutes and remove from the oven. Sprinkle crushed croutons evenly on top of each cup and return the pan to the oven for another 8-

10 minutes until the wontons are golden brown and the contents are heated through.

Crab Salad in Crisp Wonton Cup

We need variety in our diets, otherwise we get burnt out on foods we may even love and have loved for years! Chicken and beef are great, but we need an offering from the sea to round out our diet. These crab salad cups are just what you need if you're missing that taste of the ocean! Makes 18 "Cupcakes" (6 Servings) 1 Serving is 3 Cups!

NUTRITION INFORMATION PER CUP:

170 calories | 17 g carbs | 7 g fat | 9 g protein

INGREDIENTS

For the Wonton Cups:

- Cooking spray

- 18 wonton wrappers

- 2 teaspoons canola oil

- 1/4 teaspoon salt

For the Dressing:

- 1 teaspoon lime zest

- 2 tablespoons fresh lime juice

- 1/4 teaspoons salt

- 1/8 teaspoon black pepper

- 1/2 teaspoon dried hot red pepper flakes

- 2 tablespoons olive oil

For the Salad:

- 1/2 pound lump crabmeat

- 1 stalk celery

- 1/2 cup finely diced mango

- 1/4 cup thinly sliced scallions

- 2 tablespoons coarsely chopped fresh cilantro leaves

DIRECTIONS:

1. Preheat the oven to 375 degrees F. Spray 2 mini-muffin tins with cooking spray.

2. Brush the wonton wrappers with oil, and place each wrapper into a section of a mini-muffin tin. Gently press each wrapper into the tin and arrange so that it forms a cup shape. The wrapper will overlap itself and stick up out of the cup. Sprinkle with salt and bake for 8 to 10 minutes, until browned and crisp. Remove from the tin and allow wrappers to cool.

3. Meanwhile whisk together the zest, lime juice, salt, pepper, and pepper flakes. Add the oil and whisk until well combined.

4. In a medium bowl, toss together the crabmeat, celery, mango, scallions and cilantro. Add dressing and toss to combine. Fill each cup with the crab salad and serve.

Thai Chicken Salad Wonton Cups

Chicken salad can be about as fun as waiting at the DMV, are we right? Add some Thai flavor to this bland classic and you're really onto something here. Chicken can be so versatile and that is apparent in this delicious chicken salad cup. The wonton cup gives the necessary crunch to the salad. The lime and sesame seeds really give this the distinct Thai flavor you are sure to love. Makes 12 Cups.

NUTRITION INFORMATION PER CUP:

74 calories | 6.4 g carbs | 2.4 g fat | 6.2 g protein

INGREDIENTS

- 12 wonton wrappers

Dressing:

- 1 garlic, smashed
- 1½ tbsp lime juice
- 2 tsp rice vinegar
- 2½ tsp fish sauce
- 1 tsp soy sauce
- 1½ tbsp canola oil (or grape seed, vegetable or other neutral flavoured oil)
- 1 tsp sugar (or honey)

- 1 – 2 birds eye chilli, deseeded and finely chopped (or 1 – 2 tsp of chili paste or hot sauce)

Chicken Salad:

- 1½ cups shredded cooked chicken
- 1½ cups finely shredded cabbage
- ¾ cup carrot, finely julienned
- ⅓ cup finely chopped shallots/scallions

Garnish:

- Sesame seeds
- Fresh coriander/cilantro leaves

DIRECTIONS:

1. Preheat oven to 160C/320F.

2. Place wonton wrappers into a regular muffin tin, moulding it into the cups. Bake for 12 to 15 minutes, until crisp and light golden brown.

Remove from the oven and let the cups cool in the muffin tin. Store in an airtight container until required (stays crisp for up to 3 days).

3. Combine Dressing ingredients in a jar and shake to combine. Set aside for at least 10 minutes to allow the flavours to infuse.

4. Combine Chicken Salad ingredients in a bowl and toss to combine.

To serve: Discard the garlic clove from the Dressing, then toss it through the Chicken Salad. Divide the Chicken Salad between the cups. Garnish with sesame seeds and cilantro/coriander, if using. Serve immediately.

Buffalo Chicken Cups

Are buffalo wings healthy? Of course, they are not. Can we enjoy the taste of buffalo wings and still lose weight? Of course we can. This recipe takes lean chicken and delicious buffalo sauce to create a myriad of sinfully delicious flavors. These will be your new favorite over even the traditional hot wings! If you aren't a fan of blue cheese, no problem. Just substitute a couple of drops of fat free ranch dressing and there you go." Makes 24 Cups.

NUTRITION INFORMATION PER CUP:

70 calories | 4.6 g carbs | 2.7 g fat | 6.5 g protein

INGREDIENTS

- 2-3 boneless, skinless chicken breasts
- 2 Tbsp. olive oil

- 1/2 tsp. smoked paprika

- 1/2 tsp. chili powder

- 24 wonton wrappers

- 1 Tbsp. butter, melted

- 1/2 cup cayenne hot sauce

- 1/2 cup blue cheese crumbles

- 3 scallions, sliced thinly

DIRECTIONS:

1. Preheat oven to 350F degrees.

2. Brush chicken breasts with olive oil, and then sprinkle evenly with smoked paprika and chili powder. Place in a baking dish and cook for 20-30 minutes, or until the center is no longer pink and the juices run clear. Remove chicken and let cool, then shred.

3. Meanwhile, fit a wonton wrapper into each of 24 mini baking cups, pressing the wrappers carefully but firmly into sides of cups. (Be careful to keep the corners of each wonton wrapper open; otherwise you will not be able to fill them!) Bake for 5 minutes or until very lightly browned. Keep wontons in baking cups.

4. In a medium-sized bowl, stir together the melted butter and hot sauce. Add the chicken and stir until well coated. Then fill each wonton cup with a tablespoon or two of chicken, and then top with a pinch of blue cheese. Return wonton cups to oven and cook for another 5-10 minutes, or until cheese is soft and melty. Remove and top with sliced scallions, and serve warm. These are best served immediately.

Boom Bang-a-Bang Chicken Cups

Coronation Chicken is a Royal dish lin Great Brittain usually consisting of cooked chicken meat with a simple curried mayonnaise dressing. For how simple the recipe is it's kind of funny how it made its way onto the banquet menu for the coronation of Queen Elizabeth II in 1953. But it is delicious albeit simple...

These individual lettus cups embody the original essence of Coronation Chicken but in healthy single servings. Enjoy!

NUTRITION INFORMATION PER CUP:

176 calories | 6 g carbs | 10 g fat | 16 g protein

INGREDIENTS

- 100g smooth peanut butter

- 140g full-fat coconut yogurt or natural yogurt mixed with 2 tbsp desiccated coconut

- 2 tsp sweet chilli sauce

- 2 tsp soy sauce

- 2-3 spring onions finely shredded

- 3 cooked skinless chicken breasts, shredded

- 2 Baby Gem lettuces, big leaves separated

- ½ cucumber, halved lengthways, seeds scraped out with a teaspoon, cut into matchsticks

- toasted sesame seeds, for sprinkling

DIRECTIONS:

1. In your smallest pan, gently warm peanut butter, yogurt, 3 tbsp water, sweet chili and soy sauce until melted together into a smooth sauce. Set aside and allow to cool.

2. Mix the spring onions and chicken into the sauce and season. Chill until the party. Keep the lettuce leaves and cucumber under damp kitchen paper.

3. To assemble, add a bundle of cucumber to each lettuce leaf cup, plus a spoonful of the chicken mixture. Sprinkle with sesame seeds and sit on a big platter for everyone to dig in. Or simply serve a pile of lettuce leaves alongside bowls of chicken and cucumber.

Ancho Chile Ground Beef Tacos

Street tacos are normally fried in oil and contain fatty versions of meat with vegetables sauteed in oils. This makes for some seriously high-fat (small) tacos that leave you hungry and needing more food. That's no good when you're restricting calories for weight loss. Satiety and good nutrition is the name of the game.

This version of beef tacos will check all of the boxes. The use of lean ground beef and seasonings for flavor keeps the calorie count low and the flavor high.

NUTRITION INFORMATION PER TACO (4 oz.):

171 calories | 5 g carbs | 6 g fat | 25 g protein

Ingredients:

- 1 tbsp. ancho chile powder
- 1/2 tbsp. cumin
- 1/2 tsp. smoked paprika
- 1/2 tbsp. oregano
- 1/2 tbsp. garlic powder
- 1/2 tbsp. onion powder
- 1/2 tsp. coriander

- 1/2 tsp. salt

- 1/2 tsp. pepper

- 1 lb. 95% lean ground beef

- 1/3 cup water

- 1/2 tbsp. cornstarch

DIRECTIONS:

1. Mix together ancho chili powder, cumin, paprika, oregano, garlic powder, onion powder, coriander, salt, and pepper. This makes a delicious homemade taco seasoning.

2. Brown the beef (or turkey) in a skillet until cooked through. Drain any excess fat. If you like you could add vegetables during this step you could – diced onions, red and yellow peppers, canned and drained diced tomatoes, or diced zucchini would be delicious. Beans are also a delicious addition.

3. Whisk together the water and cornstarch. Add to the pan along with the taco seasoning and bring to a simmer. Let simmer for 3-4 minutes until sauce thickens.

Garlic Lemon Shrimp Kabobs

Kabobs are the ultimate single-serving food. You know exactly how much you put on the skewer and each skewer is its own serving. It doesn't get much simpler than that. Using lean shrimp makes this recipe standout because it's basically pure protein and calculable.

Add these to a salad or eat them on their own – either way, these will keep you on track with your bariatric diet!

NUTRITION PER KABOB (6 oz.):

189 calories | 2 g carbs | 7 g fat | 31 g protein

INGREDIENTS:

- 1.33 lbs shrimp, peeled and deveined

- Salt and pepper

- 2 tbsp butter, melted

- 1/4 cup freshly squeezed lemon juice

- 4 cloves garlic, minced

- 1 tsp Italian seasoning

- 2 tbsp parsley, chopped

DIRECTIONS:

1. Preheat the oven to 450 degrees or preheat the grill.

2. Add the butter to a small saucepan. Once it melts, add the garlic, lemon juice, and Italian seasoning. Cook for 2-3 minutes on low until garlic is fragrant.

3. Thread the shrimp on skewers. Season with salt and pepper. To cook in the oven, place on a baking sheet and cook for 5-6 minutes until pink and cooked through. To cook on the grill, place directly on the grill and cook for 2-3 minutes per side until opaque and cooked through.

4. When the shrimp are cooked, brush with the garlic butter mixture and serve.

Pumpkin Pie Oatmeal (with Added Protein)

Ingredients

- 1/2 Cup Nonfat Milk

- 3/4 Cup (12 TBS) Water

- 1/2 Cup Old Fashioned Oats

- Pinch Cinnamon

- Pinch Nutmeg

- 1/4 Cup Canned Pumpkin

- 2 Tbs Almond Accents Oven Roasted No Salt

- Splenda, Sugar, or Natural Sweetener to Taste

- 1/4 Cup Water

- 1 Scoop Vanilla Protein Powder

Directions

1. In small pot, bring milk and water to a boil over medium heat. Add oatmeal, cinnamon, and nutmeg. Reduce heat to medium-low and simmer until liquid is absorbed, about 7 to 15 minutes, stirring occasionally.

2. Once the liquid is absorbed, stir in pumpkin almonds, and sweetener (if desired); set aside.

3. Combine water and protein powder in a separate bowl. Mix with a fork until protein is dissolved (may be easier to use blender).

4. Pour protein mixture over oatmeal and serve.

BBQ Breakfast Chicken Burritos

Ingredients

- 4 ounces of chicken breast (i use boiled chicken breast with the bone)

- 1 tbsp Kraft barbeque sauce

- 4 egg whites

- 2 La Banderita Low Carb Low Fat Tortillas

- 1 tsp garlic powder

- 1 tsp cumin powder

- Dash of Mortons lite salt or regular salt

- 1/2 oz of Kraft 2% sharp cheddar cheese

Directions

1. First, i cook the egg whites in pam spray and add the cumin, garlic powder, and lite salt as they cook. While that is cooking, i heat up 4 oz of precooked chicken breasts and start heating up the low carb tortillas.

2. Next place half of the chicken breast in one tortilla and add 1/2 cheese, 1/2 bbq sauce, and you could add hot sauce as well.

3. Finally add the egg whites on top of this (helps melt the cheese and wrap into a burrito. You can try to add diced tomatoes, onions, and cilantro to them if you would like. I will try this next time for a Southwestern style.

4. Serves 2.

Chunky Unstuffed Green Peppers

Ingredients

- 1 lb. Ground beef, lean

- 2 large tomatoes, diced

- 2 large green peppers, diced

- 1 large onion, diced

- 1 tsp. garlic powder

- 1/2 tsp basil

- 1/2 cup rice (cooked with 1 cup of water)

Directions

1. Combine 1/2 cup rice with 1 cup of water. Cook

    per directions on rice package.

2. While rice is cooking, in large skillet, brown ground beef. Drain. Set meat aside on paper towels to continue to drain.

3. Place diced tomatoes, green peppers, onion, garlic powder, and basil in skillet. Cook on low heat for 15-20 minutes. Add ground beef and cooked rice into mixture. Salt and pepper to taste. Enjoy!

Slow Cooker Creamy Italian Chicken

Ingredients

- 2 pounds boneless, skinless chicken breasts
- 1 packet Italian dressing mix
- 1/2 cup water
- 1 (8-ounce) package reduced-fat cream cheese
- 1 can 98% fat free cream of chicken soup

- 3 cups cooked long grain rice (white or brown)

Directions

1. Place chicken in crock pot

2. Mix together Italian dressing mix and water. Pour over chicken.

3. Cover and cook on high for 4 hours OR low for 8 hours.

4. Mix together cream cheese and soup in separate bowl.

5. Carefully remove chicken from crock pot to plate.

6. Pour cream cheese/soup mixture into crock pot and mix together with dressing in bottom.

7. Return chicken to crock pot and mix gently to shred the chicken.

8. Cook on LOW until heated through.

9. Serve with rice or noodles.

Note: You may add skim or low fat milk in very small quantities to thin the sauce a little. It does not significantly affect the nutritional value if you use up to 2 tablespoons.

Slow Cooker Salsa Chicken with Cheese Soup

Ingredients

- 2 boneless, skinless chicken breast halves
- 1/2 cup salsa
- 1/2 can cheddar cheese soup or nacho cheese soup (condensed)
- 1 1/2 tsp taco seasoning
- 1/4 cup light sour cream

Directions

1. Lay chicken in bottom of 1 1/2 or 2-quart slow cooker. Sprinkle taco seasoning over chicken. Stir together salsa and cheese soup in bowl and pour over chicken. Cook on low 6-8 hours.

2. Remove stoneware from slow cooker with pot holders, take chicken out and shred with fork. Put chicken back into stoneware, then stir in sour cream. (Note: Depending on the tenderness level of your chicken, you may be able to shred it by simply stirring it inside the stoneware.)

This is great served over rice or used as an enchilada filling.

Breaded Chicken Parmesan

Ingredients

- 12 ounces white meat chicken (one double breast)
- 1 tbsp grated Parmesan cheese
- 1/4 cup Italian-style bread crumbs
- 1 tsp garlic powder
- 1 tbsp onions, dried
- Crushed red peppers if desired
- 1 -2 tbsp olive oil

Directions

1. Cut the chicken breast horizontally (filet it) so you will end up with two thin pieces.
2. Rub each piece with olive oil.
3. Mix dry ingredients together and pat each piece with the crumb mixture until well covered.

4. Bake at 375*F for about 20 minutes.

Slow-Cooker Salsa Chicken

Ingredients

- 4 boneless, skinless chicken breasts

- 1 cup salsa

- 1 package reduced sodium taco seasoning

- 1 can reduced fat cream of mushroom soup (condensed)

- 1/2 cup reduced fat sour cream

Directions

1. Add chicken to slow cooker.

2. Sprinkle taco seasoning over chicken.

3. Pour salsa and soup over chicken.

4. Cook on low for 6 to 8 hours.

5. Remove from heat and stir in sour cream.

6. Serve with rice.

Note: You may use half the packet of taco seasoning (I have started doing this to reduce sodium content myself)

Grape Salad

Ingredients

- About 2 - 4 lbs of Grapes (either Red or Green, or you can mix both is you want). Also depends on how big you want to make it.
- 1 pkg 8oz Fat Free Cream Cheese (soften)
- 1 pkg 8 oz Fat Free Sour Cream
- 1/2 c Splenda Sugar
- 4 tsps Vanilla

- 1/4 cup Brown Sugar (can use Splenda Brown Sugar)
- 1/2 cup Chopped Walnuts either Pecans

Directions

1. Wash Grape first before using and drain.
2. Mix Cream Cheese and Sour Cream, Sugar and Vanilla. Blend very well together on high for 3 -4 mins.
3. Mix Mixture and Grapes together. Thoroughly Grapes are covered.
4. Pour into a 9x13 cake pan and sprinkle with Brown Sugar lightly over mixture (may require more if needed) and then sprinkle with chopped nuts.
5. Place in frig for about 1-hour before serving.

Grape Salad

Ingredients

- About 2 - 4 lbs of Grapes (either Red or Green, or you can mix both is you want). Also depends on how big you want to make it.

- 1 pkg 8oz Fat Free Cream Cheese (soften)

- 1 pkg 8 oz Fat Free Sour Cream

- 1/2 c Splenda Sugar

- 4 tsps Vanilla

- 1/4 cup Brown Sugar (can use Splenda Brown Sugar)

- 1/2 cup Chopped Walnuts either Pecans

Directions

1. Wash Grape first before using and drain.

2. Mix Cream Cheese and Sour Cream, Sugar and Vanilla. Blend very well together on high for 3 -4 mins.

3. Mix Mixture and Grapes together. Throughly Grapes are covered.

4. Pour into a 9x13 cake pan and sprinkle with Brown Sugar lightly over mixture (may require more if needed) and then sprinkle with chopped nuts.

5. Place in frig for about 1-hour before serving.

Slow Cooker Chicken Taco Stew

Ingredients

- 1 onion, chopped

- 1 16-oz can black beans

- 1 16-oz can kidney beans

- 1 16-oz can corn (drained)

- 1 8-oz can tomato sauce

- 2 14.5-oz cans diced tomatoes w/chilies

- 1 1.25-oz packet taco seasoning

- 1-2 boneless skinless chicken breasts

Directions

1. Mix everything together in a slow cooker except chicken. Lay chicken on top and cover. Cook on low for 6-8 hours or on high for 3-4 hours. 30 minutes before serving, remove chicken and shred. Return chicken to slow cooker and stir in.

2. This is good eaten with cheese, sour cream, or tortilla chips.

Chock Full O' Flavor Chicken Salad

Ingredients

- 1.5 C grilled chicken breast, diced
- 1/4 C diced celery
- 1/4 C Craisins
- 1/2 C grapes, quartered
- 3 T Miracle Whip Light

Directions

1. Mix all ingredients together. Serve over crisp greens or as a sandwich filling.

Chock Full O' Flavor Chicken Salad

Ingredients

- C grilled chicken breast, diced
- 1/4 C diced celery
- 1/4 C Craisins
- 1/2 C grapes, quartered
- 3 T Miracle Whip Light

Directions

1. Mix all ingredients together. Serve over crisp greens or as a sandwich filling.

Amy's Mexican Chicken Casserole

Ingredients

- 2 chicken breasts, boiled and shredded
- 1 green pepper, diced

- 1 small onion, diced

- 2 cups brown rice, uncooked

- 1 16 oz. jar Red Gold Mild Salsa

- 1 10.75 oz. can Campbell's Cheddar Cheese Soup (unprepared)

- 1 15.25 oz. can yellow sweet corn, retain liquid

- 1 15 oz can black beans, rinsed and drained

- 4 Cups Water

- 1/2 Cup Shredded Cheese

Directions

1. Boil the chicken breasts in enough liquid to cover for about 15 minutes (longer if from frozen) or until they're just a little pink in the center. Shred with a fork when nearly cooked.

2. Meanwhile, dice onion and green pepper and set aside. In a really big casserole dish (I think mine is

6 quarts, and it was full!), mix 2 cups of brown rice (dry, unprepared, NOT instant), the corn and liquid in the corn can, the rinsed and drained black beans, and the cheddar cheese soup (unprepared). Add the four cups of water and stir thoroughly.

3. When the chicken's shredded, saute the onion and green pepper in a tablespoon of olive oil for a few minutes, until just soft. Then add the shredded chicken and cook 2 - 3 minutes more, until well combined and fully cooked.

4. Add the chicken mixture to the rice mixture in the big casserole dish, stir, and cover the entire thing with foil (or a lid if you have one). Cook at 400 for 1 hour, 45 minutes, stirring occasionally. Then remove foil (careful!!) and top with 1/2 cup

shredded cheddar cheese (or a blend, whatever you have...).

5. Serve with tortillas (not included in nutritional calculation).

Chicken Salad

Ingredients

- 3 lb. Chicken breast, cooked, cubed

- 3 Tbsp. Lemon juice

- 1/2 tsp. Celery seed

- 1/4 cup Kraft Miracle Whip Light

- 1 cup Light Sour Cream

- 1 cup Red Seedless Grapes, halved

- 1/4 cup Sliced Almonds

Directions

1. Boil chicken until tender; about 30 minutes. Cube and place in large bowl.

2. Add lemon juice, stir.

3. Add celery seed, stir.

4. Add Miracle whip and sour cream, stir.

5. Add grapes and almonds, stir.

6. Refrigerate for 1 hour before serving.

7. Serve with flour tortillas or crackers.

8. Makes 8 1-cup servings.

Note: You can use precooked and cubed chicken to save time if you like. You could also use fresh celery (1/2 cup) instead of the celery seed. Original recipe also calls for 1/2 cup chopped red onions.

Chicken & Grape Salad

Ingredients

- 1 pound grilled chicken

- 1 cup grapes, sliced

- 2 TBSP light mayo

- 1/4 cup walnuts

Directions

1. Mix all ingredients and serve with on lettuce or bread.

Meal Plan for Steady Weight Loss (1 Week Plan)

The 6 Daily Meal Plan can help you lose weight at a moderate rate. It is designed for anyone who is looking to lose weight, especially patients who are eating solid foods after gastric sleeve, gastric bypass, lap-band, or another type of weight loss surgery. Each day on the plan has three small high-protein meals and three high-protein snacks.

The 6 Daily Meal Plan includes:

- Lean sources of protein.
- Healthy fats and carbs.
- Quick, easy, and convenient meals and snacks.

The 6 Daily Meal Plan can help you:

- Lose weight steadily as you approach goal weight.

- Hit your protein needs each day.

- Balance the foods you eat without being restrictive or depriving yourself.

- Practice healthy habits for weight loss and long-term maintenance.

Diet Guidelines:

- Eat slowly and mindfully, and chew slowly.

- Drink plenty of water and other calorie-free or low-calorie liquids between meals to stay hydrated.

- Only use under the supervision of your doctor.

DAY 1

Breakfast

- Smoothie with ½ banana, ½ cup almond milk, 2 tablespoonsPowdered Peanut Butter, Vanilla Protein Powder (220 calories, 21 grams protein)

Snack 1

- Vanilla Cappuccino (90 calories, 15 grams protein)

Lunch

- Mini protein pizzas on with ¼ cup pizza sauce and 1 ounce mozzarella onRusk Protein Bread with any veggie toppings 1 medium pear (330 calories, 23 grams protein)

Snack 2

- Protein Potato Chips (130 calories, 10 grams protein)

Dinner

- Vegetable Chili with Beans with 1 ounce melted cheddar, 1 cup steamed cauliflower (250 calories, 23 grams protein)

Dessert

- ½ cup non-fat cottage cheese with cinnamon (90 calories, 14 grams protein)

Totals: 1110 calories, 106 grams protein

DAY 2

Breakfast

- Peaches and Cream Protein Oatmeal, ½ ounce pecans (200 calories, 16 grams protein)

Snack 1

- Proticcino Instant Protein Drink (80 calories, 15 grams protein)

Lunch

- ½ cup fat-free refried beans in roasted green pepper halves, topped with 1 ounce melted cheddar cheese (250 calories, 14 grams protein)

Snack 2

- ¼ cup roasted edamame (240 calories, 35 grams protein)

Dinner

- 4 ounces grilled chicken breast with VLC Pasta Sauce Baked sweet potato fries: 1 medium sweet potato brushed with 2 teaspoons olive oil (310 calories, 28 grams protein)

Dessert

- Baked apple with cinnamon, ½ cup sugar-free low-fat vanilla frozen yogurt (160 calories, 6 grams protein)

Totals: 1130 calories, 93 grams protein

DAY 3

Breakfast

- Strawberry Meal Replacement Shake, ½ ounce pecans (240 calories, 35 grams protein)

Snack 1

- Meat Snack Stick (70 calories, 14 grams protein)

Lunch

- Salad with romaine lettuce, tomatoes, cucumbers, 3 ounces grilled chicken, 1 ounce parmesan cheese, 2 tablespoons balsamic vinaigrette (300 calories, 33 grams protein)

Snack 2

- Chocolate Caramel Protein Granola Snacks (130 calories, 15 grams protein)

Dinner

- Eggplant Bake with ½ large eggplant in slices covered with ¼ cup fat-free ricotta, ½ cup tomato sauce, and 1 ounce mozzarella (240 calories, 14 grams protein)

Dessert

- 1 ounce dark chocolate (140 calories, 2 grams protein)

Totals: 1220 calories, 103 grams protein

DAY 4

Breakfast

- Vegetable Omelet with 1 ounce melted cheese (210 calories, 22 grams protein)

Snack 1

- Crispy Cinnamon Protein Bar (160 calories, 15 grams protein)

Lunch

- Chopped salad with lettuce, tomatoes, 3 ounces cooked shrimp or chicken, 1-ounce feta, andHoney Dijon Dressing, 1 cup sliced strawberries (280 calories, 30 grams protein)

Snack 2

- 1 cup plain Greek yogurt, 1 cup cucumber sticks (130 calories, 15 grams protein)

Dinner

- Chicken Enchilada Verde (290 calories, 10 grams protein)

Dessert

- Dulce de Leche Protein Pudding (90 calories, 15 grams protein)

Totals: 1160 calories, 107 grams protein

DAY 5

Breakfast

- Bacon and Cheese Omelet and slices of tomato on ½ whole grain, high-fiber English muffin (180 calories, 18 grams protein)

Snack 1

- ½ medium apple, sliced, 2 tablespoons peanut butter (230 calories, 8 grams protein)

Lunch

- Chicken salad lettuce wraps with 3 ounces grilled chicken breast, ½ medium diced apple, diced celery, 2 tablespoons non-fat mayo, ½ ounce walnuts on lettuce leaves (290 calories, 25 grams protein)

Snack 2

- Protein Zippers (140 calories, 15 grams protein)

Dinner

- 4 ounces broiled cod Quinoa pilaf with ½ cup quinoa (cooked in vegetable broth), ½ cup green peas, ¼ cup each diced celery and onion (330 calories, 36 grams protein)

Dessert

- Apple Cinnamon Oatmeal Cookies (110 calories, 14 grams protein)

Totals: 1280 calories, 139 grams protein

DAY 6

Breakfast

- Oatmeal Protein Bar, 1 large orange (230 calories, 14 grams protein)

Snack 1

- Aloha Mango Protein Smoothie (100 calories, 15 grams protein)

Lunch

- Cream of Tomato Protein Soup 1 slice low-calorie high-fiber bread toasted with 1 ounce swiss cheese (260 calories, 23 grams protein)

Snack 2

- 1 cup bell pepper slices, ¼ cup hummus (170 calories, 10 grams protein)

Dinner

- Low-carb tuna melt with ½ cup tuna mixed with 2 tablespoons non-fat mayo, topped with 1-ounce shredded cheddar, toasted on a portabello mushroom (250 calories, 29 grams protein)

Dessert

- Cocomint Protein Pudding (100 calories, 15 grams protein)

Totals: 1110 calories, 106 grams protein

DAY 7

Breakfast

- Honey Nut Protein Cereal with 1 container Greek yogurt and ¾ cup blueberries (270 calories, 29 grams protein)

Snack 1

- 1 cup cut melon, 1 ounce almonds (220 calories, 7 grams protein)

Lunch

- 1 cup steamed broccoli with Cheese Sauce (210 calories, 32 grams protein)

Snack 2

- 1 hard-boiled egg (80 calories, 6 grams protein)

Dinner

- 3 ounces lean ground turkey burger; mustard, sugar-free relish, ketchup; lettuce leaves, tomato slices; high-fiber bunSweet and Sour Slaw (310 calories, 23 grams protein)

Dessert

- Peanut Butter Cup Protein Bar (160 calories, 15 grams protein)

Totals: 1250 calories, 112 grams protein

The Bottom Line

While bariatric surgery is not the "easy way" as some people think, you should be enjoying life! Enjoying life to the utmost involves enjoying great-tasting food. The goal for life after bariatric surgery should be to improve your health, but also enjoying life.

Of course, the bariatric life requires discipline and commitment, so use these recipes to stay on your path to a "new you" and stay away from bland, tasteless meals!

Made in the USA
Monee, IL
17 September 2021